The Complete Diabetic Pressure Pot Cookbook

Easy and Healthy Recipes to Make Unforgettable Your Diabetic Diet

Cassandra Lane

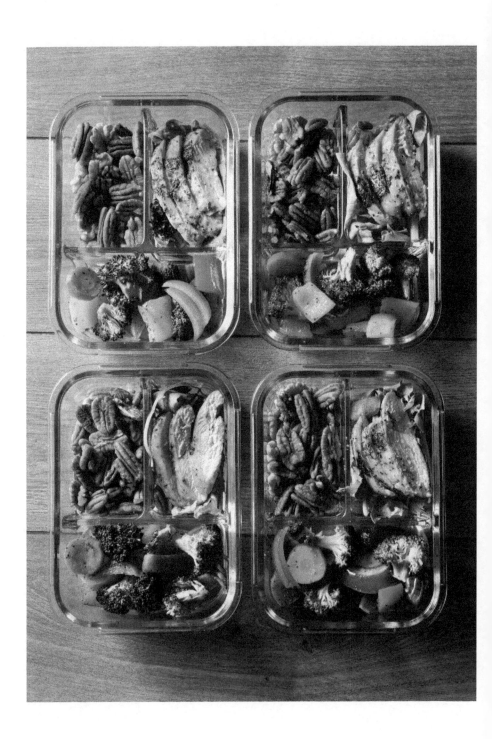

of information contained within this document, including, but not limited to, — errors, omissions, or inaccuracies.

Table of Contents

Wild Rice Salad with Cranberries and Almonds

Servings: 18

Cooking Time: 25 Minutes

Ingredients:

For the rice

- 2 cups wild rice blend, rinsed
- 1 teaspoon kosher salt
- 2½ cups Vegetable Broth or Chicken Bone Broth

For the dressing

- ¼ cup extra-virgin olive oil
- ¼ cup white wine vinegar
- 1½ teaspoons grated orange zest
- Juice of 1 medium orange (about ¼ cup)
- 1 teaspoon honey or pure maple syrup

For the salad

- ¾ cup unsweetened dried cranberries
- ½ cup sliced almonds, toasted
- Freshly ground black pepper

Directions:

1. To make the rice

2. In the electric pressure cooker, combine the rice,

salt, and broth.

3. Close and lock the lid. Set the valve to sealing.

4. Cook on high pressure for 25 minutes.

5. When the cooking is complete, hit Cancel and allow the pressure to release naturally for 1minutes, then quick release any remaining pressure.

6. Once the pin drops, unlock and remove the lid.

7. Let the rice cool briefly, then fluff it with a fork.

8. To make the dressing

9. While the rice cooks, make the dressing: In a small jar with a screw-top lid, combine the olive oil, vinegar, zest, juice, and honey. (If you don't have a jar, whisk the ingredients together in a small bowl.) Shake to combine.

10. To make the salad

11. In a large bowl, combine the rice, cranberries, and almonds.

12. Add the dressing and season with pepper.

13. Serve warm or refrigerate.

14.Nutrition Info: Per serving(⅓ CUP): Calories: 126; Total Fat: 5g; Protein: 3g; Carbohydrates: 18g; Sugars: 2g; Fiber: 2g; Sodium: 120mg.

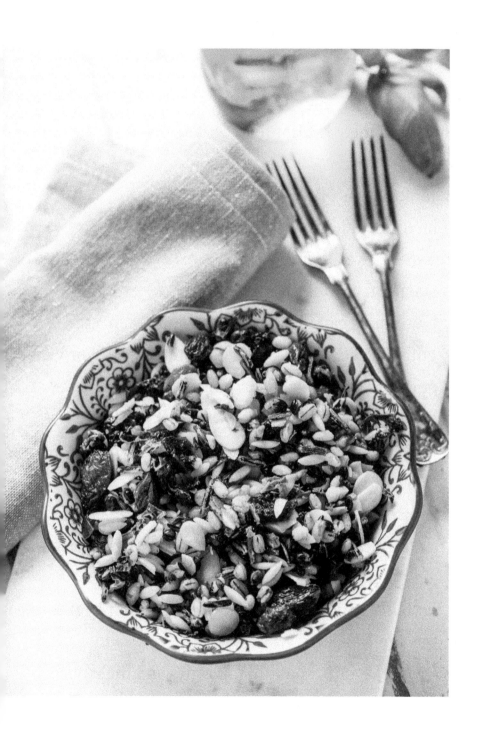

Black Bean Soup with Lime-yogurt Drizzle

Servings: 8

Cooking Time: 40 Minutes

Ingredients:

• 2 tablespoons avocado oil

• 1 medium onion, chopped

• 3 garlic cloves, minced

• 1 teaspoon ground cumin

• 1 (10-ounce) can diced tomatoes and green chilies

• 6 cups Chicken Bone Broth, Vegetable Broth, or water

• 1 pound dried black beans, rinsed

• Kosher salt

• ¼ cup plain Greek yogurt or sour cream

• 1 tablespoon freshly squeezed lime juice

Directions:

1. Set the electric pressure cooker to the Sauté setting. When the pot is hot, pour in the avocado oil.

2. Sauté the onion for 3 to 5 minutes, until it begins to soften. Hit Cancel.

3. Stir in the garlic, cumin, tomatoes and their juices, broth, and beans.

4. Close and lock the lid of the pressure cooker. Set the valve to sealing.

5. Cook on high pressure for 40 minutes.

6. While the soup is cooking, combine the yogurt and lime juice in a small bowl.

7. When the cooking is complete, hit Cancel. Allow the pressure to release naturally for 15 minutes, then quick release any remaining pressure.

8. Once the pin drops, unlock and remove the lid.

9. (Optional) For a thicker soup, remove 1½ cups of beans from the pot using a slotted spoon. Use an immersion blender to blend the beans that remain in the pot. If you don't have an immersion blender, transfer the soup left in the pot to a blender or food processor and purée. (Follow the instructions that came with your machine for blending hot foods.) Stir in the reserved beans. Season with salt, if desired.

10. Spoon into serving bowls and drizzle with lime-yogurt sauce.

11. Nutrition Info: Per serving(1 CUP): Calories: 285; Total Fat: 6g; Protein: 19g; Carbohydrates: 42g; Sugars: 3g; Fiber: 10g; Sodium: 174mg

4-Ingredient Carnitas Posole

Servings: 4

Cooking Time: 8 Minutes

Ingredients:

• 2 cups Chicken Bone Broth or low-sodium store-bought chicken broth

• 1 (15-ounce) can hominy

• 2 cups Pork Carnitas or shredded cooked pork

• 2 cups Roasted Tomatillo Salsa

• Chopped avocado, for serving (optional)

• Chopped cilantro, for garnish (optional)

Directions:

1. In the electric pressure cooker, combine the broth, hominy and its juices, pork, and salsa.
Stir to combine.

2. Close and lock the lid of the pressure cooker. Set the valve to sealing.

3. Cook on high pressure for 8 minutes.

4. When the cooking is complete, hit Cancel and quick release the pressure.

5. Once the pin drops, unlock and remove the lid.

6. Spoon into bowls and serve with avocado and/or

cilantro (if using).

7. Nutrition Info: Per serving: Calories: 264; Protein: 28g; Carbohydrates: 20g; Sugars: 5g; Fiber: 7g; Sodium: 590mg

Low Fat Roast

Servings: 2

Cooking Time: 25 Minutes.

Ingredients:

• 1lb roasting potatoes

• 1 garlic clove

• 1 cup vegetable stock

• 2tbsp olive oil

Directions:

1. Put the potatoes in the steamer basket and add the stock into the Pressure Pot.

2. Steam the potatoes in your Pressure Pot for 15 minutes.

3. Depressurize and pour away the remaining stock.

4. Set to sauté and add the oil, garlic, and potatoes. Cook until brown.

5. Nutrition Info: Per serving: Calories: 201; Carbs: 3 ; Sugar: 1 ; Fat: 6 ; Protein: 5 ; GL: 26

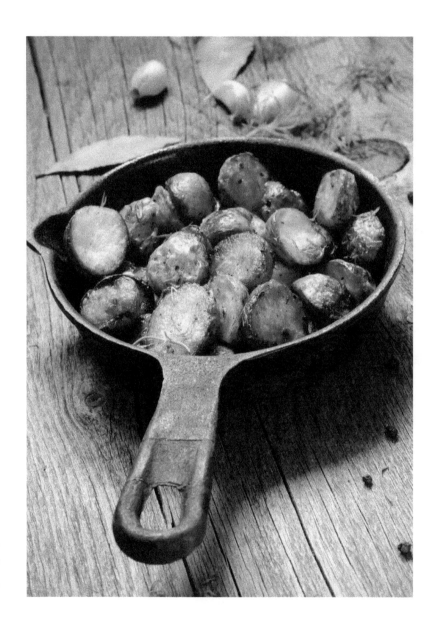

Roasted Parsnips

Servings: 2

Cooking Time: 25 Minutes.

Ingredients:

• 1lb parsnips

• 1 cup vegetable stock

• 2tbsp herbs

• 2tbsp olive oil

Directions:

1. Put the parsnips in the steamer basket and add the stock into the Pressure Pot.

2. Steam the parsnips in your Pressure Pot for 15 minutes.

3. Depressurize and pour away the remaining stock.

4. Set to sauté and add the oil, herbs and parsnips.

5. Cook until golden and crisp.

6. Nutrition Info: Per serving: Calories: 130; Carbs: 14 ; Sugar: 0 ; Fat: 0 ; Protein: 4 ; GL: 16

Lower Carb Hummus

Servings: 2

Cooking Time: 60 Minutes

Ingredients:

- 0.5 cup dry chickpeas
- 1 cup vegetable stock
- 1 cup pumpkin puree
- 2tbsp smoked paprika
- salt and pepper to taste

Directions:

1. Soak the chickpeas overnight.

2. Place the chickpeas and stock in the Pressure Pot.

3. Cook on Beans 60 minutes.

4. Depressurize naturally.

5. Blend the chickpeas with the remaining ingredients.

6. Nutrition Info: Per serving: Calories: 135;Carbs: 18 ;Sugar: 2 ;Fat: 3 ;Protein: 13 ;GL: 6

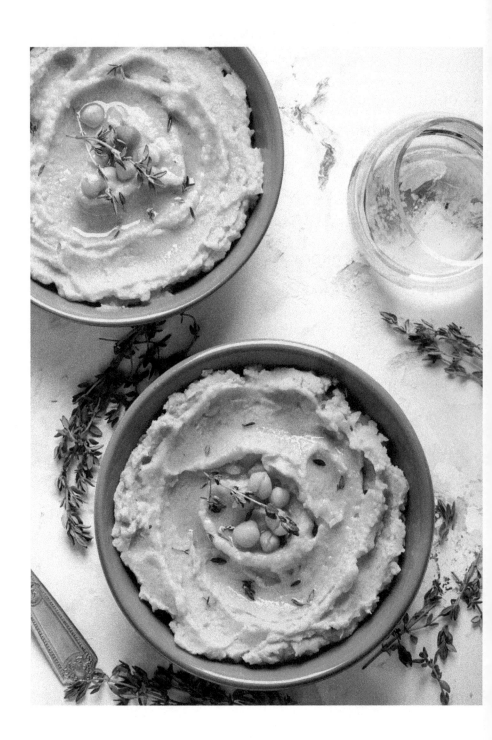

Sweet and Sour Red Cabbage

Servings: 8

Cooking Time: 10 Minutes

Ingredients:

• 2 cups Spiced Pear Applesauce or unsweetened applesauce

• 1 small onion, chopped

• ½ cup apple cider vinegar

• ½ teaspoon kosher salt

• 1 head red cabbage, cored and thinly sliced

Directions:

1. In the electric pressure cooker, combine the applesauce, onion, vinegar, salt, and cup of water. Stir in the cabbage.

2. Close and lock the lid of the pressure cooker. Set the valve to sealing.

3. Cook on high pressure for 10 minutes.

4. When the cooking is complete, hit Cancel and quick release the pressure.

5. Once the pin drops, unlock and remove the lid.

6. Spoon into a bowl or platter and serve. 7. Nutrition Info: Per serving: Calories: ; Total Fat: 0g; Protein: 2g;

Carbohydrates: 18g; Sugars: 11g; Fiber: 4g; Sodium: 160mg

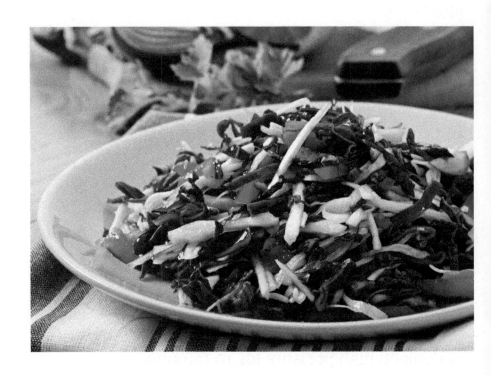

Pinto Beans

Servings: 10

Cooking Time: 55 Minutes

Ingredients:

- 2 cups pinto beans, dried
- 1 medium white onion, peeled and diced
- 1 ½ teaspoon minced garlic
- ¾ teaspoon salt
- 1/4 teaspoon ground black pepper
- 1 teaspoon red chili powder
- 1/4 teaspoon cumin
- 1 tablespoon olive oil
- 1 teaspoon chopped cilantro
- 5 ½ cup vegetable stock

Directions:

1. Plugin Pressure Pot, insert the inner pot, press sauté/simmer button, add oil and when hot, add onion and garlic and cook for 3 minutes or until onions begin to soften.

2. Add remaining ingredients, stir well, then press the cancel button, shut the Pressure Pot with its lid and turn the pressure knob to seal the pot.

3. Press the „manual" button, then press the „timer" to set the cooking time to 45 minutes and cook at high pressure, Pressure Pot will take 5 minutes or more for building its inner pressure.

4. When the timer beeps, press „cancel" button and do natural pressure release for 10 minutes until pressure nob drops down.

5. Open the Pressure Pot, spoon beans into plates and serve.

6. Nutrition Info: Calories: .1 Cal, Carbs: 11.7 g, Fat: 0.2 g, Protein: 3.7 g, Fiber: 4 g.

Parmesan Cauliflower Mash

Servings: 4

Cooking Time: 5 Minutes

Ingredients:

• 1 head cauliflower, cored and cut into large florets

• ½ teaspoon kosher salt

• ½ teaspoon garlic pepper

• 2 tablespoons plain Greek yogurt

• ¾ cup freshly grated Parmesan cheese

• 1 tablespoon unsalted butter or ghee (optional)

• Chopped fresh chives

Directions:

1. Pour cup of water into the electric pressure cooker and insert a steamer basket or wire rack.

2. Place the cauliflower in the basket.

3. Close and lock the lid of the pressure cooker. Set the valve to sealing.

4. Cook on high pressure for 5 minutes.

5. When the cooking is complete, hit Cancel and quick release the pressure.

6. Once the pin drops, unlock and remove the lid.

7. Remove the cauliflower from the pot and pour out

the water. Return the cauliflower to the pot and add the salt, garlic pepper, yogurt, and cheese. Use an immersion blender or potato masher to purée or mash the cauliflower in the pot.

8. Spoon into a serving bowl, and garnish with butter (if using) and chives.

9. Nutrition Info: Per serving: Calories: 141; Total Fat: 6g; Protein: 12g; Carbohydrates: 12g; Sugars: 5g; Fiber: 4g; Sodium: 5mg

Chili Greens

Servings: 2

Cooking Time: 10 Minutes

Ingredients:

• 2 cups mixed cabbage, shredded

• 1 cup trimmed green beans

• 3 stalks chopped scallions

• 2tbsp chili paste

• salt and pepper to taste

Directions:

1. Mix the ingredients in the Pressure Pot.

2. Seal and cook on Stew for 10 minutes. Depressurize naturally.

3. Nutrition Info: Per serving: Calories: 60;Carbs: 12 ;Sugar: 1 ;Fat: 0 ;Protein: 2 ;GL: 4

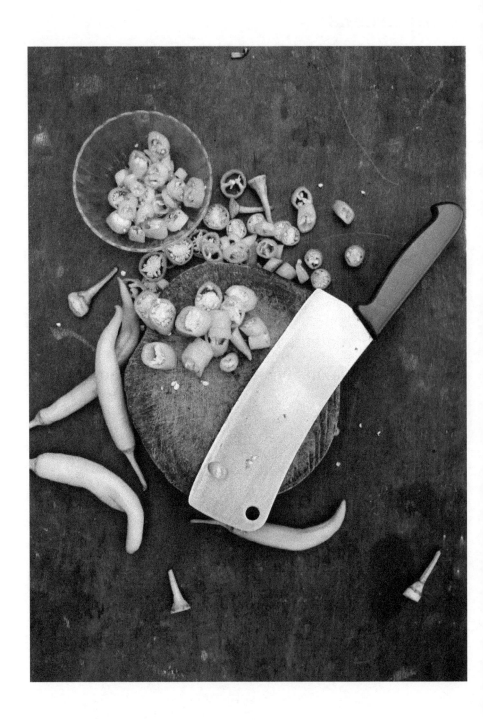

Hummus Dahl

Servings: 2

Cooking Time: 60 Minutes

Ingredients:

- 0.5 cup dry lentils
- 0.5 cup pumpkin puree
- 1 cup vegetable stock
- 2tbsp light tahini

Directions:

1. Soak the lentils overnight.

2. Place the lentils and stock in the Pressure Pot.

3. Cook on Beans 60 minutes.

4. Depressurize naturally.

5. Blend the lentils with the remaining ingredients.

6. Nutrition Info: Per serving: Calories: 135;Carbs: 14 ;Sugar: 1 ;Fat: 10 ;Protein: 15 ;GL: 5

Carrot and Swede

Servings: 2

Cooking Time: 15 Minutes

Ingredients:

- 1 cup chopped carrots
- 1 cup chopped swede
- 1 cup vegetable broth
- 2tbsp minced garlic

Directions:

1. Place the ingredients in your Pressure Pot.

2. Seal and cook on Stew 15 minutes.

3. Strain any excess broth.

4. Mash the carrots and swede until the texture is as desired.

5. Nutrition Info: Per serving: Calories: 60;Carbs: 10 ;Sugar: 1 ;Fat: 1 ;Protein: 2 ;GL: 1

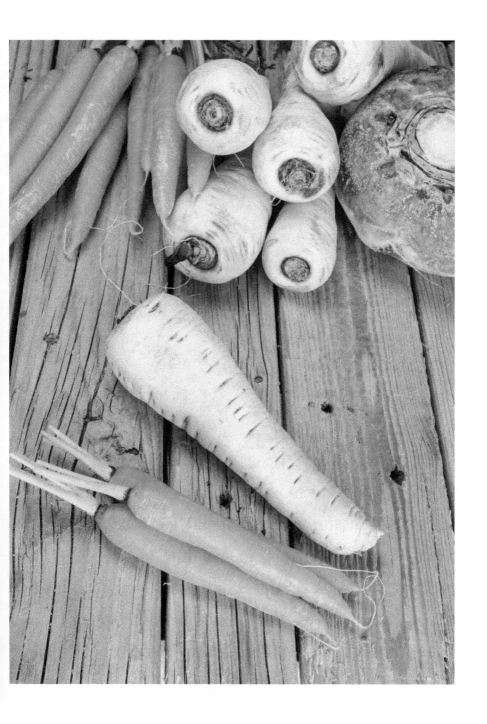

Lemon Hummus

Servings: 6

Cooking Time: 40 Minutes

Ingredients:

- 1-pound chickpeas, dried
- 2 lemons, juiced
- 1 tablespoon chopped parsley
- 1 teaspoon minced garlic
- 1/8 teaspoon salt
- 2 tablespoons olive oil
- 1/4 cup tahini paste
- 1/2 of lemon, zested
- 12 cups water

Directions:

1. Plugin Pressure Pot, insert the inner pot, add chickpeas, and pour in water.

2. Shut the Pressure Pot with its lid, turn the pressure knob to seal the pot, press the „manual" button, then press the „timer" to set the cooking time to 35 minutes and cook at high pressure, Pressure Pot will take 5 minutes or more for building its inner pressure.

3. When the timer beeps, press „cancel" button and do

natural pressure release for 10 minutes and then do quick pressure release until pressure nob drops down.

4. Open the Pressure Pot, drain chickpeas, and transfer to a food processor.

5. Add remaining ingredients except for lemon zest and parsley and pulse chickpeas for 1 to 2 minutes or until smooth, frequently scraping the sides of a food processor.

6. Add water if the hummus is too thick, then tip it in a bowl and garnish with lemon zest and parsley.

7. Serve straight away.

8. Nutrition Info: Calories: 70 Cal, Carbs: 4 g, Fat: 5 g, Protein: 2 g, Fiber: 1 g.

Honey Parsnips

Servings: 2

Cooking Time: 15 Minutes

Ingredients:

- 1lb parsnips, peeled and chopped into fingers
- 3tbsp white or rose wine
- 3tbsp butter
- 2tbsp rosemary
- 1tbsp honey
- 1tbsp balsamic vinegar

Directions:

1. Place the parsnips in your Pressure Pot with butter and parsnips and rosemary, put on Sauté until brown.

2. Add the honey, wine, and balsamic.

3. Sauté until thick and syrupy.

4. Nutrition Info: Per serving: Calories: 135;Carbs: 17 ;Sugar: 13 ;Fat: 7 ;Protein: 2 ;GL: 17

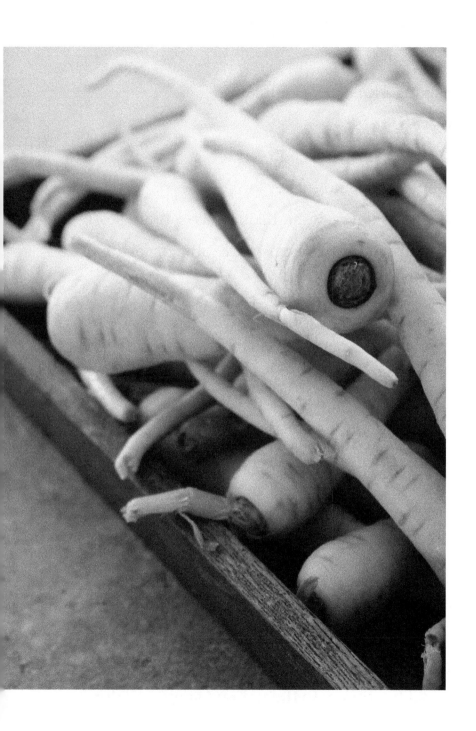

Turkey Barley Vegetable Soup

Servings: 8

Cooking Time: 20 Minutes

Ingredients:

• 2 tablespoons avocado oil

• 1 pound ground turkey

• 4 cups Chicken Bone Broth, low-sodium store-bought chicken broth, or water • 1 (28-ounce) carton or can diced tomatoes

• 2 tablespoons tomato paste

• 1 (15-ounce) package frozen chopped carrots (about 2½ cups)

• 1 (15-ounce) package frozen peppers and onions (about 2½ cups)

• ⅓ cup dry barley

• 1 teaspoon kosher salt

• ¼ teaspoon freshly ground black pepper

• 2 bay leaves

Directions:

1. Set the electric pressure cooker to the Sauté/More setting. When the pot is hot, pour in the avocado oil.

2. Add the turkey to the pot and sauté, stirring

frequently to break up the meat, for about 7 minutes or until the turkey is no longer pink. Hit Cancel.

3. Add the broth, tomatoes and their juices, and tomato paste. Stir in the carrots, peppers and onions, barley, salt, pepper, and bay leaves.

4. Close and lock the lid of the pressure cooker. Set the valve to sealing.

5. Cook on high pressure for 20 minutes.

6. When the cooking is complete, hit Cancel and allow the pressure to release naturally for 10 minutes, then quick release any remaining pressure.

7. Once the pin drops, unlock and remove the lid. Discard the bay leaves.

8. Spoon into bowls and serve.

9. Nutrition Info: Per serving(1¼ CUP): Calories: 253; Total Fat: 12g; Protein: 1; Carbohydrates: 21g; Sugars: 7g; Fiber: 7g; Sodium: 560mg

Lemony Brussels Sprouts with Poppy Seeds

Servings: 4

Cooking Time: 2 Minutes

Ingredients:

- 1 pound Brussels sprouts
- 2 tablespoons avocado oil, divided
- 1 cup Vegetable Broth or Chicken Bone Broth
- 1 tablespoon minced garlic
- ½ teaspoon kosher salt
- Freshly ground black pepper
- ½ medium lemon
- ½ tablespoon poppy seeds

Directions:

1. Trim the Brussels sprouts by cutting off the stem ends and removing any loose outer leaves.
Cut each in half lengthwise (through the stem).

2. Set the electric pressure cooker to the Sauté/More setting. When the pot is hot, pour in 1
tablespoon of the avocado oil.

3. Add half of the Brussels sprouts to the pot, cut side down, and let them brown for to 5

minutes without disturbing. Transfer to a bowl and add the remaining tablespoon of avocado

 oil and the remaining Brussels sprouts to the pot. Hit Cancel and return all the Brussels

 sprouts to the pot.

4. Add the broth, garlic, salt, and a few grinds of pepper. Stir to distribute the seasonings.

5. Close and lock the lid of the pressure cooker. Set the valve to sealing.

6. Cook on high pressure for 2 minutes.

7. While the Brussels sprouts are cooking, zest the lemon, then cut it into quarters. 8. When the cooking is complete, hit Cancel and quick release the pressure.

9. Once the pin drops, unlock and remove the lid.

10. Using a slotted spoon, transfer the Brussels sprouts to a serving bowl. Toss with the lemon

 zest, a squeeze of lemon juice, and the poppy seeds. Serve immediately.

11. Nutrition Info: Per serving: Calories: 125; Total Fat: 8g; Protein: 4g; Carbohydrates: 13g;

 Sugars: 3g; Fiber: 5g; Sodium: 504mg

Tomato Ketchup

Servings: 6

Cooking Time: 20 Minutes

Ingredients:

• 50-ounce tomatoes, quartered

• 2 mushrooms, diced

• 1/4 teaspoon onion powder

• 2 teaspoons powdered erythritol

• 1/4 teaspoon garlic powder

• 1/4 teaspoon allspice

• 4 tablespoons white vinegar

Directions:

1. Plugin Pressure Pot, insert the inner pot, add all the ingredients, and stir until mixed.

2. Shut the Pressure Pot with its lid, turn the pressure knob to seal the pot, press the „manual" button, then press the „timer" to set the cooking time to 10 minutes and cook at high pressure, Pressure Pot will take 5 minutes or more for building its inner pressure.

3. When the timer beeps, press „cancel" button and do natural pressure release for 10 minutes and then do quick pressure release until pressure nob drops down.

4. Open the Pressure Pot, puree the mixture until smooth and then press „sauté/simmer" button to cook ketchup for 5 minutes or until thickened to desired consistency.

5. When done, ladle ketchup into a jar, let cool completely and serve.

6. Nutrition Info: Calories: 14 Cal, Carbs: 3.g, Fat: 0.1 g, Protein: 0.2 g, Fiber: 0.8 g.

Spaghetti Squash

Servings: 4

Cooking Time: 7 Minutes

Ingredients:

• 1 spaghetti squash (about 2 pounds)

Directions:

1. Cut the spaghetti squash in half crosswise and use a large spoon to remove the seeds.

2. Pour 1 cup of water into the electric pressure cooker and insert a wire rack or trivet.

3. Place the squash halves on the rack, cut side up.

4. Close and lock the lid of the pressure cooker. Set the valve to sealing.

5. Cook on high pressure for 7 minutes.

6. When the cooking is complete, hit Cancel and quick release the pressure.

7. Once the pin drops, unlock and remove the lid.

8. With tongs, remove the squash from the pot and transfer it to a plate. When it is cool enough to handle, scrape the squash with the tines of a fork to remove the strands. Discard the skin.

9. Nutrition Info: Per serving: Calories: 10; Total Fat:

0g; Protein: 0g; Carbohydrates: 3g; Sugars: 1g; Fiber: 1g; Sodium: 17mg

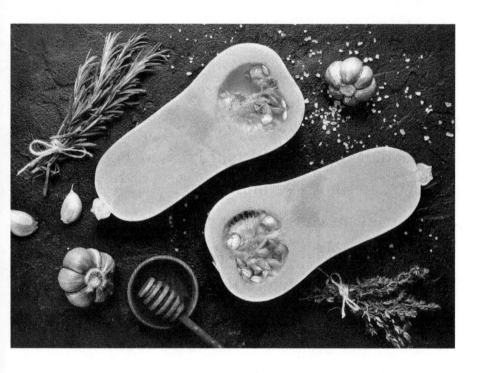

Irish Stew

Servings: 2

Cooking Time: 35 Minutes

Ingredients:

- 1.5lb diced lamb shoulder
- 1lb chopped vegetables
- 1 cup low sodium beef broth
- 3 minced onions
- 1tbsp ghee

Directions:

1. Mix all the ingredients in your Pressure Pot.

2. Cook on Stew for 35 minutes.

3. Release the pressure naturally.

4. Nutrition Info: Per serving: Calories: 330;Carbs: 9 ;Sugar: 2 ;Fat: 12 ;Protein: ;GL: 3

Taco Soup

Servings: 4

Cooking Time: 15 Minutes

Ingredients:

- 1 tbsp. olive oil
- 1 diced yellow onion
- 2 minced garlic cloves
- 15 oz. drained black beans
- 14 oz. crushed tomatoes
- 1 cup frozen sweetcorn
- 3 diced bell peppers
- 6 cups vegetable broth
- 1 box chickpea pasta shells
- 1 sliced jalapeño pepper, sliced
- 1 tbsp. chili powder
- 1 tsp. ground cumin
- 1 tsp. dried oregano
- ½ tsp. sea salt

To Serve:

- Fresh cilantro
- 1 sliced avocado

Directions:

1. Add the olive oil, onions, garlic, tomatoes, corn, beans, spices and vegetable broth to instant Pot. Stir gently.

2. Cover and seal the lid, making sure the steam release valve is set to "Sealing."

3. Cook on the "Manual, High Pressure" setting for minutes, and once done, do a quick release of the pressure.

4. Stir in the diced bell peppers and chickpeas pasta, and then sit for 5-10 minutes.

5. Ladle the soup into bowls, top with the diced jalapeño, fresh cilantro and sliced avocados, and then serve.

6. Nutrition Info: Calories 430, Carbs 74g, Fat 9g, Protein 27g, Potassium (K) 0 mg, Sodium (Na) 921 mg

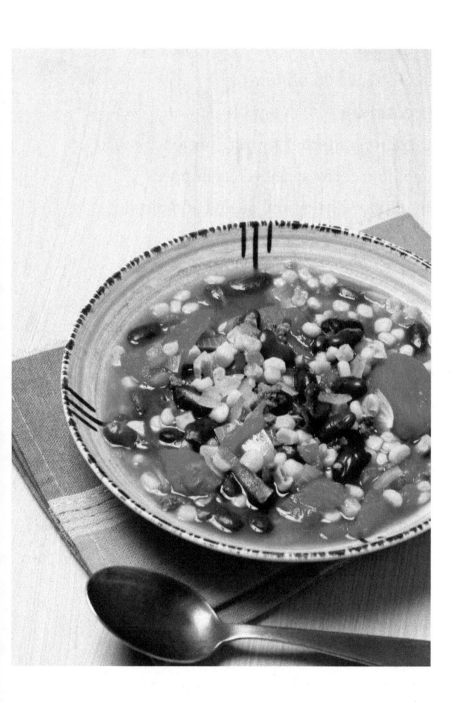

Butternut Squash and Carrot Soup

Servings: 6

Cooking Time: 20 Minutes

Ingredients:

- 1 medium butternut squash, peeled & cubed
- 3 medium carrots, peeled & chopped
- 1 medium white onion, peeled and diced
- 1 teaspoon minced garlic
- 1 tablespoon grated ginger
- 2 cups vegetable broth
- 1 tablespoon curry powder
- 1/2 teaspoon garam masala
- 1/4 teaspoon turmeric powder
- 1 teaspoon salt
- 1/4 teaspoon cayenne
- 1 lime, juiced

Directions:

1. Plugin Pressure Pot, insert the inner pot, add all the ingredients, and stir until mixed.

2. Shut the Pressure Pot with its lid and turn the pressure knob to seal the pot.

3. Press the „manual" button, then press the „timer" to

set the cooking time to 15 minutes and cook at high pressure, Pressure Pot will take 5 minutes or more for building its inner pressure.

4. When the timer beeps, press „cancel" button and do quick pressure release until pressure nob drops down.

5. Open the Pressure Pot, stir the soup and ladle into serving bowls.

6. Drizzle soup with lime juice and serve.

7. Nutrition Info: Calories: 166 Cal, Carbs: 19 g, Fat: 10 g, Protein: 2 g, Fiber: 3 g.

Chicken Stew

Servings: 6

Cooking Time: 16 Minutes

Ingredients:

- 2 (6-ounce) boneless, skinless chicken breasts
- ½ cup brown rice, rinsed
- ½ cup dried lentils
- 1 large, sweet potato, peeled and cubed
- 3½ cups water
- 2 tablespoons olive oil
- 4 garlic cloves, minced
- 1 teaspoon ground coriander
- 1 teaspoon ground cumin
- ½ teaspoon ground coriander
- 1 teaspoon cayenne pepper
- Salt and ground black pepper, as required

Directions:

1. In the Pressure Pot, place oil and press "Sauté". Now add the chicken and cook for about 4-5 minutes or until browned completely.

2. With a slotted spoon, transfer the chicken breasts onto a plate.

3. In the pot, add the garlic and cook for about 1 minute.

4. Press "Cancel" and sir in the remaining ingredients.

5. Close the lid and place the pressure valve to "Seal" position.

6. Press "Manual" and cook under "High Pressure" for about 10 minutes.

7. Press "Cancel" and carefully allow a "Quick" release.

8. Open the lid and with tongs, transfer the chicken breasts onto a cutting board

9. With a knife, cut the chicken into bite-sized pieces.

10. Add the chicken pieces into the pot and stir to combine.

11. Serve hot.

12. Nutrition Info: Per serving: Calories: 289, Fats: 9.6g, Carbs: 27.8g, Sugar: 2g, Proteins: 22.5g, Sodium: 88mg

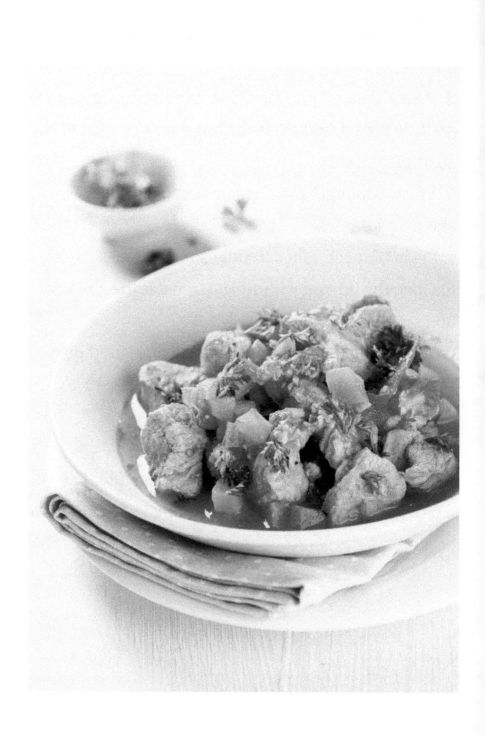

Sweet and Sour Soup

Servings: 2

Cooking Time: 35 Minutes

Ingredients:

- 1lb cubed chicken breast
- 1lb chopped vegetables
- 1 cup low carb sweet and sour sauce
- 0.5 cup diabetic marmalade

Directions:

1. Mix all the ingredients in your Pressure Pot.

2. Cook on Stew for 35 minutes.

3. Release the pressure naturally.

4. Nutrition Info: Per serving: Calories: 270;Carbs: 22 ;Sugar: 9 ;Fat: 2 ;Protein: 36 ;GL: 12

Egg Salad

Servings: 4

Cooking Time: 5 Minutes

Ingredients:

• 8 eggs

• ¼ cup celery, diced

• ⅓ cup homemade mayonnaise

• 1 tsp. sea salt

• ½ tsp. black pepper

• Cooking oil spray

Directions:

1. Lightly spray a baking or casserole dish with cooking oil spray and crack the eggs into the dish.

2. Place a wire steamer rack in the bottom of the Pressure Pot and add a cup of water.

3. Place the baking dish on the rack and seal the Pressure Pot lid.

4. Cook on the "Manual, High Pressure" setting for 5 minutes, and then release the steam manually when the cook cycle completes.

5. Remove the baking dish from the pot and slide the egg loaf onto a cutting board.

6. Chop and then combine with mayonnaise, celery, salt, and black pepper.

7. Chill until ready to serve.

8. Nutrition Info: Calories 266, Carbs 5.3g, Fat 22g, Protein 11g, Potassium (K) 137 mg, Sodium (Na) 714 mg

Pumpkin Soup

Servings: 2

Cooking Time: 10 Minutes

Ingredients:

• 1 lb. chopped pumpkin

• 1 lb. chopped tomato

• 1 cup broth

• 1tbsp. mixed herbs

• 1 minced onion

Directions:

1. Mix all the ingredients in your Pressure Pot.

2. Cook on Stew for 10 minutes.

3. Release the pressure naturally.

4. Blend.

5. Nutrition Info: Calories 200, Carbs 7g, Fat 11g, Protein 2g, Potassium (K) 2 mg, Sodium (Na) 1033 mg

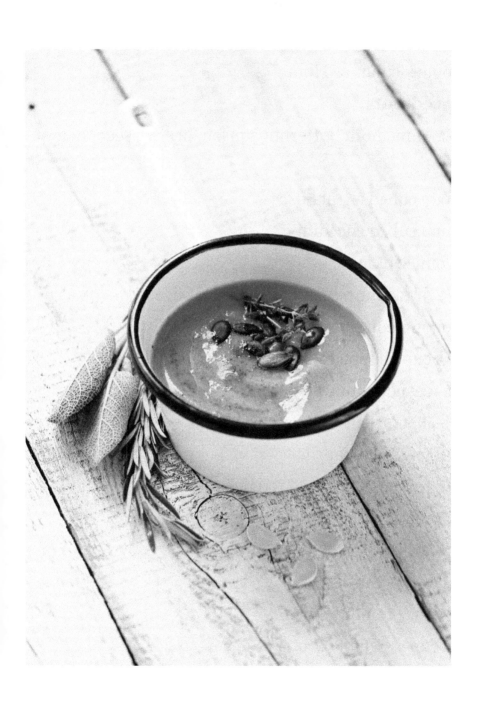

Mediterranean Stew

Servings: 5

Cooking Time: 10 Hours

Ingredients:

• 1/2 of medium butternut squash, peeled, seeded, and cubed

• 1 cup cubed eggplant

• 1 cup cubed zucchini

• 5-ounce okra

• 1/2 of medium carrot, peeled and sliced

• 1/2 of medium tomato, chopped

• 1/2 cup chopped white onion

• ½ teaspoon minced garlic

• 1 teaspoon salt

• 1/8 teaspoon paprika

• 1/8 teaspoon crushed red pepper

• 1/8 teaspoon ground turmeric

• 1/4 teaspoon ground cumin

• 2 tablespoons raisins

• 4-ounce tomato sauce

• ½ cup vegetable broth

Directions:

1. Plugin Pressure Pot, insert the inner pot, add all the ingredients, and stir until mixed.

2. Press the cancel button, shut the Pressure Pot with its lid and turn the pressure knob to seal the pot.

3. Press the „slow cook" button, then press the „timer" to set the cooking time to 10 hours at low heat setting.

4. When the timer beeps, press „cancel" button and do natural pressure release for until pressure nob drops down.

5. Open the Pressure Pot, then ladle stew into bowls and serve.

6. Nutrition Info: Calories: 122 Cal, Carbs: 30.5 g, Fat: 0.5 g, Protein: 3.4 g, Fiber: 8 g.

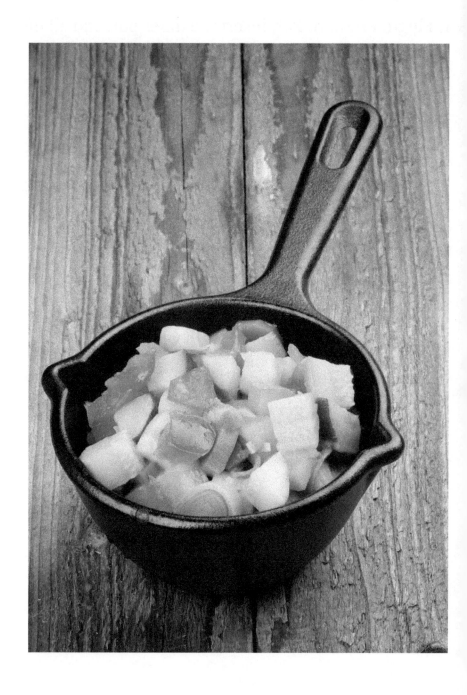

Rutabaga Stew

Servings: 6

Cooking Time: 25 Minutes

Ingredients:

- 2 medium rutabagas, peeled and diced
- 1 stalk of celery, diced
- 2 medium beets, peeled and diced
- 2 medium carrots, peeled and diced
- ½ of small red onion, peeled and diced
- 1 teaspoon salt
- 1/3 teaspoon ground black pepper
- 1 1/4 teaspoons olive oil
- 2 ½ cups chicken stock

Directions:

1. Plugin Pressure Pot, insert the inner pot, press sauté/simmer button, add oil and when hot, add celery, onion, and garlic and cook for 5 minutes or until tender.

2. Add remaining ingredients, stir until mixed, then press the cancel button, shut the Pressure Pot with its lid and turn the pressure knob to seal the pot.

3. Press the „manual" button, then press the „timer" to

set the cooking time to 15 minutes and cook at high
pressure, Pressure Pot will take 5 minutes or more for
building its inner pressure.

4. When the timer beeps, press „cancel" button and do
quick pressure release until pressure nob drops down.

5. Open the Pressure Pot, stir the soup and then puree
using an immersion blender until smooth.

6. Ladle soup into bowls and serve.

7. Nutrition Info: Calories: 85.3 Cal, Carbs: 12.9 g, Fat:
2.1 g, Protein: 3.g, Fiber: 3.9 g.

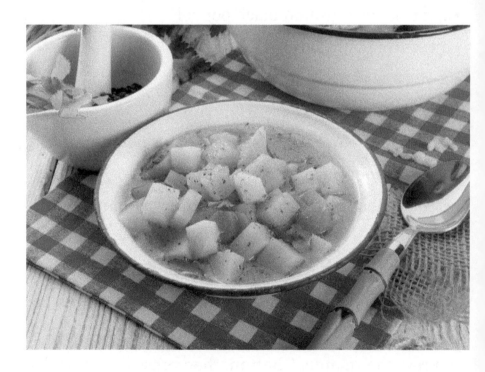

Cream of Tomato Soup

Servings: 2

Cooking Time: 15 Minutes

Ingredients:

- 1lb fresh tomatoes, chopped
- 1.5 cups low sodium tomato puree
- 1tbsp black pepper

Directions:

1. Mix all the ingredients in your Pressure Pot.

2. Cook on Stew for 15 minutes.

3. Release the pressure naturally.

4. Blend.

5. Nutrition Info: Per serving: Calories: 20;Carbs: 2 ;Sugar: 1 ;Fat: 0 ;Protein: 3 ;GL: 1

Shiitake Soup

Servings: 2

Cooking Time: 35 Minutes

Ingredients:

- 1 cup shiitake mushrooms
- 1 cup diced vegetables
- 1 cup low sodium vegetable broth
- 2tbsp 5 spice seasoning

Directions:

1. Mix all the ingredients in your Pressure Pot.

2. Cook on Stew for 35 minutes.

3. Release the pressure naturally.

4. Nutrition Info: Per serving: Calories: 70;Carbs: 5 ;Sugar: 1 ;Fat: 2 ;Protein: 2 ;GL: 1

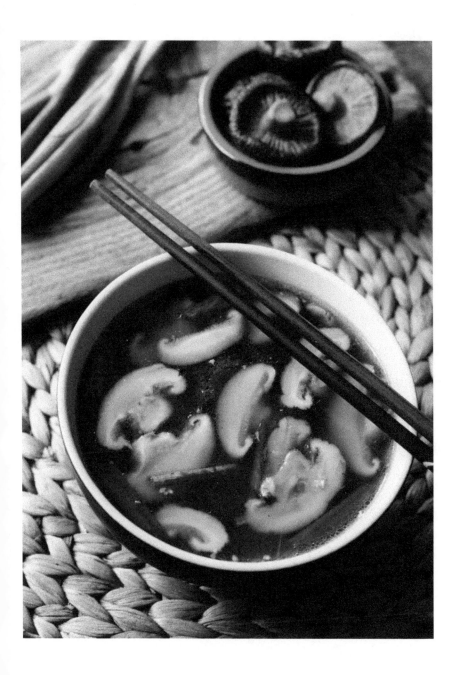

Chili con Carne

Servings: 2

Cooking Time: 35 Minutes

Ingredients:

- 1lb minced beef
- 1 cup mixed beans
- 2 cups chopped tomatoes
- 3 squares very dark chocolate
- 3tbsp mixed seasoning

Directions:

1. Mix all the ingredients in your Pressure Pot.

2. Cook on Stew for 35 minutes.

3. Release the pressure naturally.

4. Nutrition Info: Per serving: Calories: 3;Carbs: 16 ;Sugar: 6 ;Fat: 12 ;Protein: 46 ;GL: 14

Broccoli Stilton Soup

Servings: 2

Cooking Time: 35 Minutes

Ingredients:

• 1lb chopped broccoli

• 0.5lb chopped vegetables

• 1 cup low sodium vegetable broth

• 1 cup Stilton

Directions:

1. Mix all the ingredients in your Pressure Pot.

2. Cook on Stew for 35 minutes.

3. Release the pressure naturally.

4. Blend the soup.

5. Nutrition Info: Per serving: Calories: 280;Carbs: 9 ;Sugar: 2 ;Fat: 22 ;Protein: 13 ;GL: 4

Irish Beef Stew

Servings: 4

Cooking Time: 35 Minutes

Ingredients:

- 1-pound beef, cut into 1-inch pieces
- 1 large white onion, peeled and diced
- 2 stalks of celery, sliced
- 2 medium potatoes, cut into 1-inch pieces
- 2 medium carrots, peeled and sliced
- 1 teaspoon minced garlic
- 1 teaspoon salt
- 1/2 teaspoon ground black pepper
- 1 teaspoon dried thyme
- 1 tablespoon dried parsley
- 1 bay leaf
- 1 tablespoon olive oil
- 1 cup beef stock
- 2 tablespoons cornstarch
- 2 tablespoons warm water

Directions:

1. Plugin Pressure Pot, insert the inner pot, press sauté/simmer button, add oil and when hot, add onion,

celery, carrot, and garlic and cook for 5 minutes or until softened.

2. Add remaining ingredients, except for cornstarch and warm water, stir until mixed and press the cancel button.

3. Shut the Pressure Pot with its lid, turn the pressure knob to seal the pot, press the „manual" button, then press the „timer" to set the cooking time to 20 minutes and cook at high pressure, Pressure Pot will take 5 minutes or more for building its inner pressure.

4. When the timer beeps, press „cancel" button and do natural pressure release for 10 minutes and then do quick pressure release until pressure nob drops down.

5. Open the Pressure Pot, stir together cornstarch and water, add into the stew, stir well and let stew rest for minutes or until slightly thick.

6. Ladle stew into the bowls and serve.

7. Nutrition Info: Calories: 392.8 Cal, Carbs: 61.6 g, Fat: 4.1 g, Protein: 29.1 g, Fiber: 9.8 g.

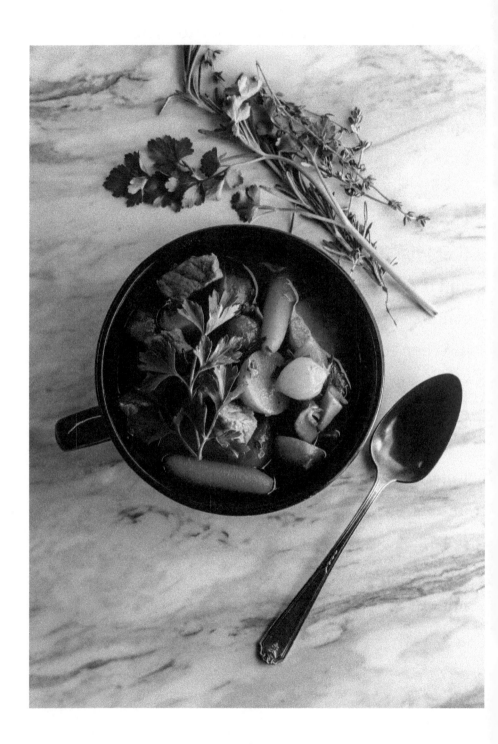

Beef & Green Beans Soup

Servings: 4

Cooking Time: 38 Minutes

Ingredients:

• 1 pound lean ground beef

• 1 cup fresh tomatoes, chopped finely

• ½ pound fresh green beans, trimmed and cut into 1-inch pieces

• 1 medium onion, chopped

• 4 cups low-sodium beef broth

• 1 tablespoon olive oil

• 1 tablespoon garlic, minced

• 2 teaspoons dried thyme, crushed

• 1 teaspoon ground cumin

• Ground black pepper, as required

Directions:

1. In the Pressure Pot, place oil and press "Sauté". Now add the beef and cook for about 5 minutes or until browned completely.

2. Add the onion, garlic, thyme, cumin and cook for about 3 minutes.

3. Press "Cancel" and stir in the tomatoes, beans and

broth.

4. Close the lid and place the pressure valve to "Seal" position.

5. Press "Manual" and cook under "Low Pressure" for about 30 minutes.

6. Press "Cancel" and carefully allow a "Quick" release.

7. Open the lid and stir in the black pepper.

8. Serve hot.

9. Nutrition Info: Per serving: Calories: 2, Fats: 10.9g, Carbs: 9g, Sugar: 3.2g, Proteins: 39.4g, Sodium: 533mg

Broccoli Soup

Servings: 6

Cooking Time: 15 Minutes

Ingredients:

• 1 small yellow onion, chopped

• 3 scallions, chopped

• 1¾ pounds broccoli florets

• 5½ cups low-sodium chicken broth

• 2 tablespoon olive oil

• Ground black pepper, as required

Directions:

1. In the Pressure Pot, place oil and press "Sauté". Now add the onion, scallion, curry powder and cook for about 5 minutes.

2. Add the broccoli and cook for about minutes

3. Press "Cancel" and stir in the broth.

4. Close the lid and place the pressure valve to "Seal" position.

5. Press "Manual" and cook under "High Pressure" for about minutes.

6. Press "Cancel" and allow a "Natural" release for about 10 minutes. Then allow a "Quick" release.

7. Open the lid and with an immersion blender, puree the soup.

8. Press "Sauté" and stir in black pepper.

9. Cook for about 2-3 minutes.

10.Press "Cancel" and serve hot.

11. Nutrition Info: Per serving: Calories: 106, Fats: 5.1g, Carbs: 4g, Sugar: 2.9g, Proteins: 5.8g, Sodium: 109mg

Kidney Bean Stew

Servings: 2

Cooking Time: 15 Minutes

Ingredients:

• 1lb cooked kidney beans

• 1 cup tomato passata

• 1 cup low sodium beef broth

• 3tbsp Italian herbs

Directions:

1. Mix all the ingredients in your Pressure Pot.

2. Cook on Stew for 15 minutes.

3. Release the pressure naturally.

4. Nutrition Info: Per serving: Calories: 270;Carbs: 16 ;Sugar: 3 ;Fat: 10 ;Protein: 23 ;GL: 8

White Beans & Rice Curry

Servings: 8

Cooking Time: 1½ Hours

Ingredients:

• 2 cups dry white beans, soaked for 8 hours and drained

• 2 cups brown rice, rinsed

• 1 sweet potato, peeled and sliced

• ½ onion, chopped

• 10 cups water

• 2 garlic cloves, minced

• Salt and ground black pepper, as required

• 1 tablespoon curry powder

• 1 teaspoon red pepper flakes, crushed

• 1 teaspoon ground coriander

• ½ teaspoon ground cumin

Directions:

1. In the pot of Pressure Pot, place all ingredients and mix well.

2. Close the lid and place the pressure valve to "Seal" position.

3. Press "Stew" and just use the default time of 90

minutes.

4. Press "Cancel" and allow a "Natural" release.

5. Open the lid and serve hot.

6. Nutrition Info: Per serving: Calories: 253, Fats: 1.5g, Carbs: 45g, Sugar: 1.8g, Proteins: 8.1g, Sodium: 54mg

DESSERT

Hot Chocolate

Servings: 2

Cooking Time: 2 Minutes

Ingredients:

• 4tbsp double cream

• 6tsp powdered sweetener

• 3tsp sugar-free cocoa

• 1/4tsp vanilla extract

• hot water or fat-free milk

Directions:

1. Mix all the ingredients in your Pressure Pot.

2. Seal and cook on Stew for minutes.

3. Depressurize naturally.

4. Stir well and serve.

5. Nutrition Info: Per serving: Calories: 100;Carbs: 3 ;Sugar: 1 ;Fat: 11 ;Protein: 4 ;GL: 1

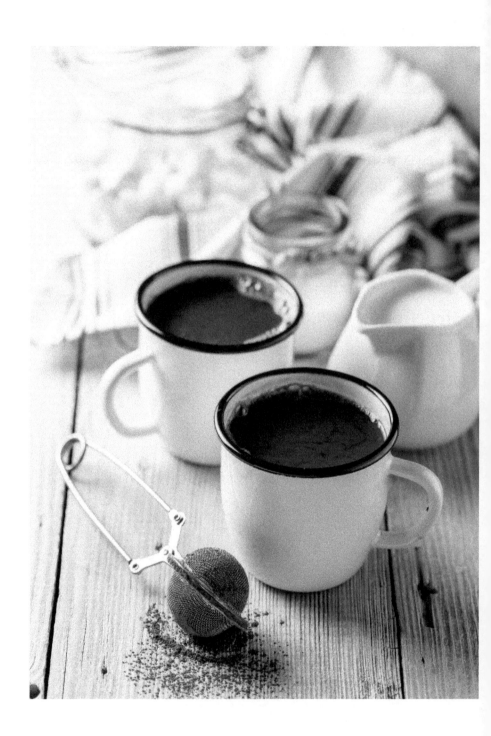

Molten Brownie Cups

Servings: 4

Cooking Time: 10 Minutes

Ingredients:

- ⅔ cup sugar-free or paleo-friendly chocolate chips
- 3½ tbsps. almond flour
- ⅔ cup Swerve granular sweetener
- 6 tbsps. salted butter
- 3 beaten eggs
- 1 tsp. pure vanilla extract

Directions:

1. Grease four 6-ounce ramekins with coconut oil spray and set aside for now.

2. Melt together sugar-free chocolate chips and butter over medium-low heat. Remove and set aside.

3. Combine the eggs, almond flour, sweetener, and vanilla extract in a medium bowl. Whisk thoroughly.

4. Pour the melted butter and chocolate into the egg and flour mixture and thoroughly whisk to combine.

5. Fill each ramekin halfway with the batter.

6. Add 1¾ cup of water to the Pressure Pot and place a steamer rack into the pot.

7. Place three of the four ramekins onto the rack and stack the fourth ramekin in the center stacked on top of the other three ramekins.

8. Close and seal the lid, making sure the steam release handle in the "Sealing" position.

9. Select the "Pressure Cook" or the "Manual, High Pressure" setting and adjust to cook for minutes.

10. Once done, using oven mitts turn the steam release handle to "Venting" and then do a quick pressure release.

11. Once all the steam is released, carefully open the lid and remove the ramekins.

12. Cool for 5 - 7 minutes, and then serve warm, topped with sugar- free whipped cream if you like.

13. Nutrition Info: Calories 425, Carbs 11g, Fat 36g, Protein 9 g, Potassium (K) 170 mg, Sodium (Na) 210 mg

Pumpkin Oatmeal

Servings: 2

Cooking Time: 5 Minutes

Ingredients:

- 1/4 cup oats
- 1 cup milk
- 1 cup pumpkin puree
- 4tbsp sweetener
- 1tsp cinnamon

Directions:

1. Pour the milk into your Pressure Pot.

2. Add the remaining ingredients, stir well. Seal and close the vent.

3. Choose Manual and set to cook 5 minutes. Release the pressure naturally.

4. Nutrition Info: Per serving: Calories: 320;Carbs: 1;Sugar: 2 ;Fat: 2 ;Protein: 3 ;GL: 5

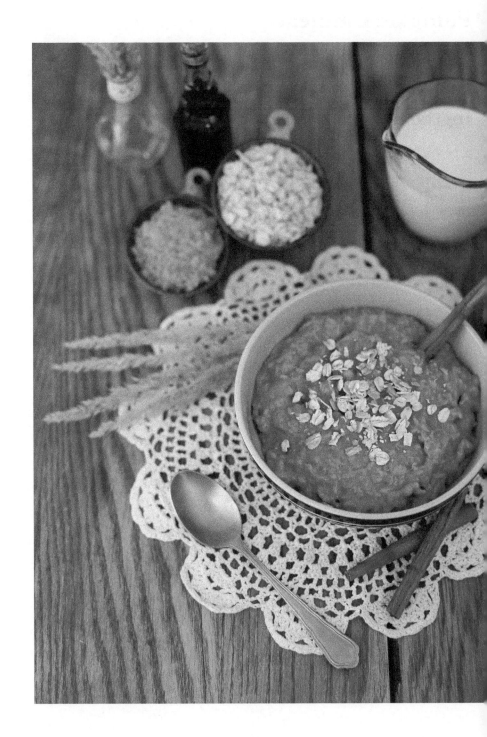

Chocolate Fudge

Servings: 8

Cooking Time: 10 Minutes

Ingredients:

- 2 1/2 cups chocolate chips, unsweetened
- 1/8 teaspoon salt
- 2 teaspoons liquid stevia, vanilla flavored
- 1 teaspoon vanilla extract, unsweetened
- 1/3 cup coconut milk, reduced fat

Directions:

1. Plugin Pressure Pot, insert the inner pot, add all the ingredients, stir until just mixed, then press the „sauté/simmer" button and whisk the mixture until well combined.

2. Press the cancel button, press the „keep warm" button, and continue whisking the mixture until all chocolate chips are well melted.

3. Take a rimmed baking sheet, lined with aluminum foil, then grease with oil and pour in chocolate mixture.

4. Place the baking sheet into the refrigerator and chill for hours or more until firm.

5. Cut fudge into square pieces and serve.

6. Nutrition Info: Calories: 90 Cal, Carbs: 18 g, Fat: 3 g, Protein: 0.5 g, Fiber: 0.4 g.

Mixed Berries Compote

Servings: 4

Cooking Time: 8 Minutes

Ingredients:

• 2 cups fresh mixed berries, divided

• ½ cup Erythritol

• 1 tablespoon arrowroot starch

• 1 tablespoon water

• 2 tablespoons fresh lemon juice

Directions:

1. In the pot of Pressure Pot, place cups of berries, Erythritol and lemon juice and stir to combine.

2. Close the lid and place the pressure valve to "Seal" position.

3. Press "Manual" and cook under "High Pressure" for about minutes.

4. Press "Cancel" and allow a "Natural" release for about 10 minutes. Then allow a "Quick" release.

5. Meanwhile, in a small bowl, dissolve arrowroot starch in water.

6. Open the lid and press "Sauté".

7. Add the arrowroot starch mixture and stir to

combine.

8. Cook for about 4-5 minutes, stirring continuously.

9. Stir in remaining berries and Press "Cancel".

10. Transfer compote into a bowl and keep aside in room temperature to cool completely.

11. Refrigerate before serving.

12. Nutrition Info: Per serving: Calories: 49, Fats: 0.3g, Carbs: 10.4g, Sugar: 5.2g, Proteins: 0.6g, Sodium: 2mg

Zucchini Pudding

Servings: 4

Cooking Time: 10 Minutes

Ingredients:

• 2 cups zucchini, shredded

• 10 ounces unsweetened almond milk

• ¼ cup Erythritol

• ½ teaspoon ground cardamom

Directions:

1. In the pot of Pressure Pot, place all ingredients except cardamom and stir to combine.

2. Close the lid and place the pressure valve to "Seal" position.

3. Press "Manual" and cook under "High Pressure" for about 10 minutes.

4. Press "Cancel" and allow a "Natural" release for about 10 minutes. Then allow a "Quick" release.

5. Open the lid and stir in cardamom.

6. Transfer the pudding into a serving bowl and refrigerate to chill before serving.

7. Nutrition Info: Per serving: Calories: 21, Fats: 1.1g, Carbs: 2.6g, Sugar: 1g, Proteins: 1g, Sodium: 5g

Lime Curd

Servings: 3

Cooking Time: 15 Minutes

Ingredients:

• 2 teaspoons grated lime zest

• 1 cup swerve sweetener

• 2/3 cup lime juice

• 2 eggs

• 2 egg yolks

• 3-ounce butter, soften

• 1 ½ cup water

Directions:

1. Place butter and sweetener in a bowl and beat for 2 minutes or until fluffy.

2. Then beat in eggs and egg yolks for 1 minute or until blended and then stir in lime juice until combined.

3. Plugin Pressure Pot, insert the inner pot, pour in water, and insert a steamer basket.

4. Divide curd mixture evenly between three half-pint mason jars and place lids on them.

5. Place mason jars on the steamer basket, shut the Pressure Pot with its lid and turn the pressure knob to

seal the pot.

6. Press the „manual" button, then press the „timer" to set the cooking time to 10 minutes and cook at high pressure, Pressure Pot will take 5 minutes or more for building its inner pressure.

7. When the timer beeps, press „cancel" button and do natural pressure release for 10 minutes and then do quick pressure release until pressure nob drops down.

8. Open the Pressure Pot, remove mason jars, then open carefully and stir lime zest into curd until mixed.

9. Close jars with the lid tightly and then cool in the refrigerator for 4 hours or overnight or until curd get thick.

10. Serve straight away.

11. Nutrition Info: Calories: 45 Cal, Carbs: 8 g, Fat: 1 g, Protein: 1 g, Fiber: 0 g.

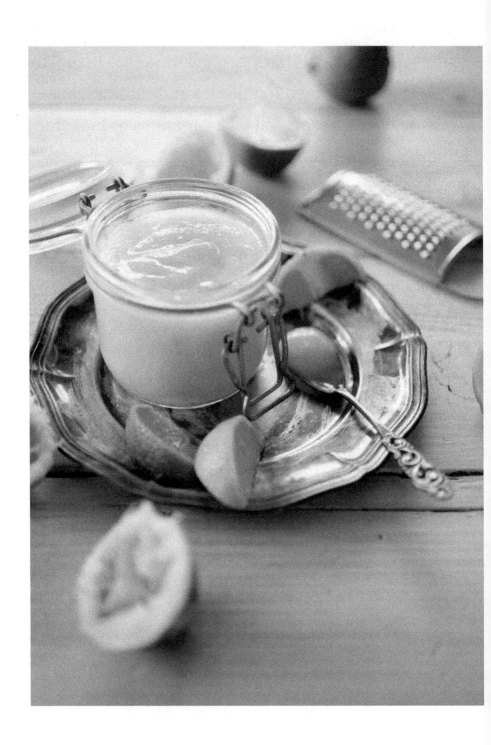

Vanilla Mug Cake

Servings: 2

Cooking Time: 10 Minutes

Ingredients:

- ¾ cup almond flour
- 2 eggs
- 2 tablespoons yacon syrup
- 1 teaspoon organic vanilla extract Pinch of salt

Directions:

1. In a bowl, place all the ingredients and stir to combine.

2. Divide the mixture into (8-ounce) greased mason jars evenly.

3. With a piece of foil, cover each jar.

4. Arrange a steamer trivet in the Pressure Pot and pour 1 cup of water.

5. Place the jars on top of trivet.

6. Close the lid and place the pressure valve to "Seal" position.

7. Press "Manual" and cook under "High Pressure" for about 10 minutes.

8. Press "Cancel" and carefully allow a "Quick" release.

9. Open the lid and serve warm.

10. Nutrition Info: Per serving: Calories: 364, Fats: 26.9g, Carbs: 14.1g, Sugar: 5.6g, Proteins: 5.5g, Sodium: 146mg.

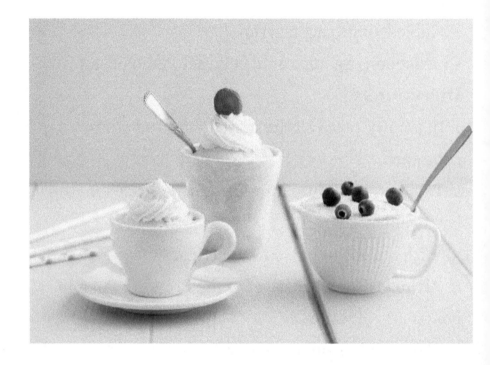

Yogurt Custard

Servings: 5

Cooking Time: 20 Minutes

Ingredients:

- 1 cup fat-free plain Greek yogurt
- 2 cups unsweetened almond milk
- ½ cup Erythritol
- 2 teaspoons ground cardamom

Directions:

1. In a heatproof pan, place all the ingredients and mix well.

2. With a piece of foil, cover the pan completely.

3. Put a steamer trivet in the bottom of Pressure Pot and pour 1 cup of water.

4. Place the pan on top of trivet.

5. Close the lid and place the pressure valve to "Seal" position.

6. Press "Manual" and cook under "High Pressure" for about 20 minutes.

7. Press "Cancel" and allow a "Natural" release for about 10 minutes. Then allow a "Quick" release.

8. Open the lid of Pressure Pot and set aside to cool.

9. Refrigerate to chill before serving.

10. Nutrition Info: Per serving: Calories: 46, Fats: 1.6g, Carbs: 3.4g, Sugar: 0.6g, Proteins: 5.3g, Sodium: 95mg

Crustless Key Lime Cheesecake

Servings: 8

Cooking Time: 35 Minutes

Ingredients:

• Nonstick cooking spray

• 16 ounces light cream cheese (Neufchâtel), softened

• ⅔ cup granulated erythritol sweetener

• ¼ cup unsweetened Key lime juice (I like Nellie & Joe's Famous Key West Lime Juice)

• ½ teaspoon vanilla extract

• ¼ cup plain Greek yogurt

• 1 teaspoon grated lime zest

• 2 large eggs

• Whipped cream, for garnish (optional)

Directions:

1. Spray a 7-inch springform pan with nonstick cooking spray. Line the bottom and partway up the sides of the pan with foil.

2. Put the cream cheese in a large bowl. Use an electric mixer to whip the cream cheese until smooth, about minutes. Add the erythritol, lime juice, vanilla, yogurt, and zest, and blend until smooth. Stop the mixer and

scrape down the sides of the bowl with a rubber spatula. With the mixer on low speed, add the eggs, one at a time, blending until just mixed. (Don't overbeat the eggs.)

3. Pour the mixture into the prepared pan. Drape a paper towel over the top of the pan, not touching the cream cheese mixture, and tightly wrap the top of the pan in foil. (Your goal here is to keep out as much moisture as possible.)

4. Pour 1 cup of water into the electric pressure cooker.

5. Place the foil-covered pan onto the wire rack and carefully lower it into the pot.

6. Close and lock the lid of the pressure cooker. Set the valve to sealing.

7. Cook on high pressure for 35 minutes.

8. When the cooking is complete, hit Cancel. Allow the pressure to release naturally for 20 minutes, then quick release any remaining pressure.

9. Once the pin drops, unlock and remove the lid.

10. Using the handles of the wire rack, carefully transfer the pan to a cooling rack. Cool to room temperature, then refrigerate for at least 3 hours.

11. When ready to serve, run a thin rubber spatula around the rim of the cheesecake to loosen it, then remove the ring.

12. Slice into wedges and serve with whipped cream (if using).

13. Nutrition Info: Per serving(1 SLICE): Calories: 157; Total Fat: 12g; Protein: 8g; Carbohydrates: 4g; Sugars: 1g; Fiber: 0g; Sodium: 196mg.

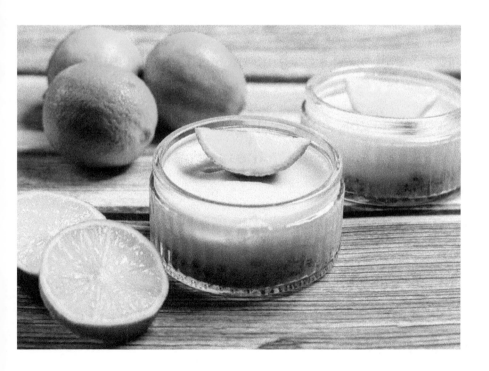

Goat Cheese–stuffed Pears

Servings: 4

Cooking Time: 2 Minutes

Ingredients:

• 2 ounces goat cheese, at room temperature

• 2 teaspoons pure maple syrup

• 2 ripe, firm pears, halved lengthwise and cored

• 2 tablespoons chopped pistachios, toasted

Directions:

1. Pour cup of water into the electric pressure cooker and insert a wire rack or trivet.

2. In a small bowl, combine the goat cheese and maple syrup.

3. Spoon the goat cheese mixture into the cored pear halves. Place the pears on the rack inside the pot, cut side up.

4. Close and lock the lid of the pressure cooker. Set the valve to sealing.

5. Cook on high pressure for 2 minutes.

6. When the cooking is complete, hit Cancel and quick release the pressure.

7. Once the pin drops, unlock and remove the lid.

8. Using tongs, carefully transfer the pears to serving plates.

9. Sprinkle with pistachios and serve immediately.

10. Nutrition Info: Per serving(½ PEAR): Calories: 120; Total Fat: 5g; Protein: 4g; Carbohydrates: 17g; Sugars: 11g; Fiber: 3g; Sodium: 54mg

Tapioca Berry Parfaits

Servings: 4

Cooking Time: 6 Minutes

Ingredients:

- 2 cups unsweetened almond milk
- ½ cup small pearl tapioca, rinsed and still wet
- 1 teaspoon almond extract
- 1 tablespoon pure maple syrup
- 2 cups berries
- ¼ cup slivered almonds

Directions:

1. Pour the almond milk into the electric pressure cooker. Stir in the tapioca and almond extract.

2. Close and lock the lid of the pressure cooker. Set the valve to sealing.

3. Cook on High pressure for 6 minutes.

4. When the cooking is complete, hit Cancel. Allow the pressure to release naturally for 10 minutes, then quick release any remaining pressure.

5. Once the pin drops, unlock and remove the lid. Remove the pot to a cooling rack.

6. Stir in the maple syrup and let the mixture cool for

about an hour.

7. In small glasses, create several layers of tapioca, berries, and almonds. Refrigerate for 1 hour.

8. Serve chilled.

9. Nutrition Info: Per serving(6 TABLESPOONS TAPIOCA, ½ CUP BERRIES, AND 1 TABLESPOON ALMONDS): Calories: 174; Total Fat: 5g; Protein: 3g; Carbohydrates: 32g; Sugars: 11g; Fiber: 3g; Sodium: 77mg

Chocolate Pudding

Servings: 4

Cooking Time: 35 Minutes

Ingredients:

• 4 ounces unsweetened chocolate, chopped

• 1 tablespoon cocoa powder, unsweetened

• 1 teaspoon salt

• 1/3 cup brown sugar

• 1 teaspoon Vanilla extract, unsweetened

• 4 egg yolks

• 1 1/2 cups whipping cream, reduced fat

• 1 ¼ cups water

Directions:

1. Place a saucepan over medium heat, add cream and heat for 3 to 4 minutes or until hot.

2. Then remove the pan from heat, add chocolate, then stir until chocolate melts and smooth mixture comes together.

3. Beat in remaining ingredients, except for water, and then strain the chocolate mixture into a round baking dish that fits into the Pressure Pot.

4. Plugin Pressure Pot, insert the inner pot, pour in

water, and insert trivet stand.

5. Cover baking dish with aluminum foil, then place it on trivet stand, press the cancel button, shut the Pressure Pot with its lid and turn the pressure knob to seal the pot.

6. Press the „manual" button, then press the „timer" to set the cooking time to 22 minutes and cook at low pressure, Pressure Pot will take 5 minutes or more for building its inner pressure.

7. When the timer beeps, press „cancel" button and do natural pressure release for 5 minutes and then do quick pressure release until pressure nob drops down.

8. Open the Pressure Pot, remove baking dish and uncover it and let cool at room temperature.

9. Cover the baking dish and chill in the refrigerator for 4 hours or overnight and then serve.

10. Nutrition Info: Calories: 120 Cal, Carbs: 21 g, Fat: 3.5 g, Protein: 1 g, Fiber: 1 g.

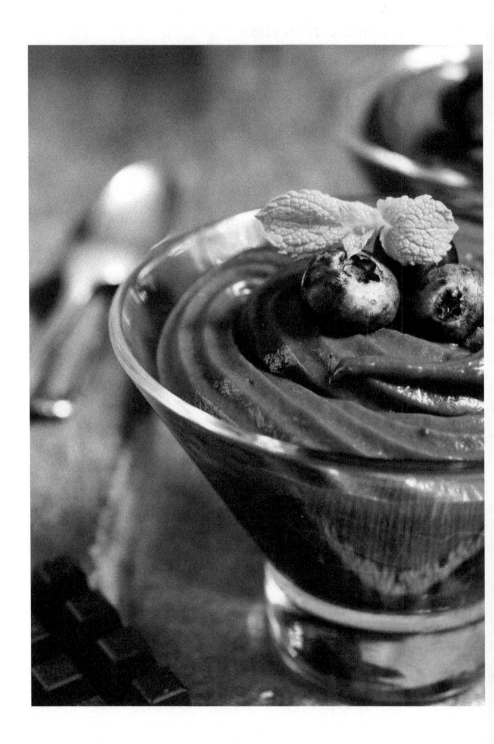

Apple Crunch

Servings: 4

Cooking Time: 2 Minutes

Ingredients:

• 3 apples, peeled, cored, and sliced (about 1½ pounds)

• 1 teaspoon pure maple syrup

• 1 teaspoon apple pie spice or ground cinnamon

• ¼ cup unsweetened apple juice, apple cider, or water

• ¼ cup low-sugar granola

Directions:

1. In the electric pressure cooker, combine the apples, maple syrup, apple pie spice, and apple juice.

2. Close and lock the lid of the pressure cooker. Set the valve to sealing.

3. Cook on high pressure for 2 minutes.

4. When the cooking is complete, hit Cancel and quick release the pressure.

5. Once the pin drops, unlock and remove the lid.

6. Spoon the apples into 4 serving bowls and sprinkle each with 1 tablespoon of granola.

7. Nutrition Info: Per serving: Calories: 103; Total Fat:

1g; Protein: 1g; Carbohydrates: 26g; Sugars: 18g; Fiber: 4g; Sodium: 13mg.

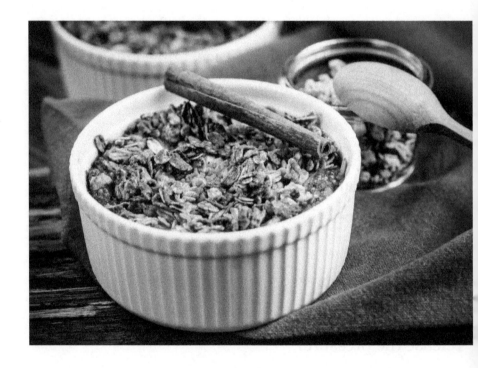

Lightning Source UK Ltd.
Milton Keynes UK
UKHW020624190721
387392UK00001B/6